Color My Yoga

Working with Chakra Energy to Lose Weight

by Cheri Haüg

www.ColorMyYoga.com
© 2017 Cheri Haüg

The material contained in this book is not intended as medical advice. If you have a medical issue or illness, consult a qualified physician.

Introduction

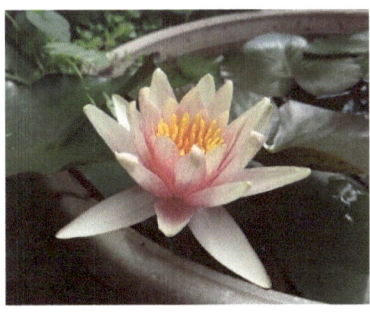 If you've ever been to a yoga studio or picked up a book about yoga, you will recognize the symbol of the lotus (pictured). The lotus starts its journey from seed to blossom in the mud at the bottom of a pond. The plant grows up through the mud and up through the water. When it surfaces into the light it becomes a beautiful flower. In this book you will learn how yoga can help you transform into your best self. Yoga can provide amazing and valuable tools to use in your weight loss journey.

Let me begin by saying that I do not believe in dieting. Dieting is a sure way to *gain* weight! Research shows that 90% of diets fail.[1] And when people do lose weight, 90 to 95% of people are unable to keep the weight off long-term.[2] Researchers have found that people on diets typically lose 5 to 10 percent of their starting weight in the first six months. However, at least one-third to two-thirds of people on diets regain more weight than they lost within four or five years, and the true number may well be significantly higher.[3] Studies also indicate that dieting is actually a consistent predictor of future weight gain. One study found that both men and women who participated in formal weight-loss programs gained significantly more weight over a two-year period than those who had not participated in a weight-loss program.[4]

The easiest way to lose weight and the surest way to keep it off is by giving up old unhealthy habits and replacing them with new healthier habits.[5] It is in this aspect of losing weight that yoga can help you.

To incorporate new healthier habits into your life, choose only one bad habit at a time and work on it for 4 weeks. After that, focus on another problem area for the next 4 weeks. You might forgo your evening dish of ice cream, the bag of chips in front of the television or your daily trip to the fast food drive-up. An easy way to approach weight loss is to reduce your daily calorie consumption by 500 calories. This can lead to a loss of one pound a week.[6] You might also try creating new habits like exercising once or twice a week. Maybe you can sign up for a yoga class or make a habit of walking or bike riding. Take baby steps in your transformation to avoid overwhelming your willpower.

This book will show you how yoga can help you make these changes and transform into a healthier new you!

I've deliberately kept this book small so that you can carry it with you as a handy reference when your willpower starts to fail you. Feel free to write in the margins and tab sections of the book that resonate with your weight loss struggles.

Yoga is for Everybody and Every Body

In our society, yoga has a reputation for being all about skinny young women in spandex.[7] I call them "the pretty people." People who are overweight or who are over the age of say, 45 or 50, often think that they don't belong in a yoga class and that they won't fit in. They think they won't be able to twist themselves into a pretzel. Men don't want to do yoga because they think it is a girl thing. The fact is that even though TV commercials often show the pretty people doing yoga, in reality, practically everybody is doing yoga now. Of course there are advanced classes with the pretty people in their size zero spandex twisting themselves into knots. But a quick phone call to any yoga studio will reveal that classes are being offered for beginners, seniors, pregnant women, the disabled, children and everybody in between.

Another notion I would like to dispel about yoga is that it is nothing more than an exercise program that helps you stretch. Yoga can be so much more. The word, "yoga" means "yoke" or "union." Yoga is in its essence about the union between mind and body. We will explore this mind body connection with the help of pranayama breathing, chakra energy centers, meditation, mudra hand gestures and more.

Yoga Asana Practice and Weight Loss

It seems that we hear about new research on the benefits of yoga almost weekly. Study after study proves what yogis have always known; that yoga provides many benefits to health, wellness, fitness and emotional well-being. It is a fact that yoga makes you stronger, builds and tones muscles, improves flexibility and improves mobility. It helps you cope with stress and it just plain feels good.

The American Council on Exercise (ACE) recently studied the physical benefits of yoga and found that "the regular practice of Hatha yoga significantly improved the subjects' flexibility, muscular strength and endurance, and balance. After eight weeks, the average flexibility of the [study participants] improved by 13% to 35% ... Similarly, the yoga [participants'] muscular strength and endurance was also boosted by regular Hatha yoga."[8]

The word "asana" means "posture" in Sanskrit. When most people think of yoga, they picture people stretching and exercising in yoga poses (asanas) like downward facing dog. This physical exercise dimension of yoga is also referred to as "Hatha." Hatha yoga, the most widely practiced form of yoga in the West, focuses on strength, balance and flexibility while coordinating breath to movement. There are other types of yoga that are more spiritual or focused more on meditation.

Yoga Builds Muscle to Help You Burn More Calories

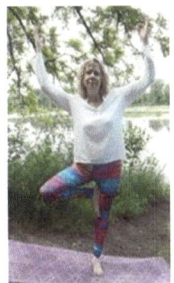 When you consider yoga purely as a form of exercise, such as Hatha yoga, you will find that it has much to offer. It helps improve your balance when you do tree pose (pictured) and it helps you get more flexible when you do forward fold (toe touches). But a lot of people who have never tried yoga don't realize how much it helps to tone and strengthen the muscles. For example, warrior poses build your leg muscles and downward facing dog works your arm muscles.

Your metabolism is a function of how quickly you burn calories when you are at rest. The surest way to boost your metabolism is by increasing your muscle mass. While you are exercising, you naturally burn more calories than when you are at rest. But after exercise, you go back to your basal metabolic rate or resting caloric burn. By increasing your muscle mass, you burn more calories at rest, i.e., you increase your basal metabolism. Muscle burns more calories than fat and increasing your muscle mass increases your daily calorie expenditure. This is the reason, in general, that men require more calories than women. They naturally carry a larger percentage of muscle mass than women and benefit from a correspondingly higher metabolism.

By building your muscles with yoga, it stands to reason that you can increase your metabolism to burn more calories and ultimately lose some weight.

Yoga Is a Gateway to More Vigorous Forms of Exercise

To increase your rate of weight loss, you need to engage in more strenuous exercise than what is offered in an average Hatha yoga class.

As an exercise program, yoga improves several important components of physical fitness: flexibility, muscular endurance, muscular strength, agility and coordination.

Basic Hatha yoga classes are missing the element of aerobic conditioning.[9] Aerobic exercise provides two big benefits. 1. It improves your cardiorespiratory fitness making your heart and lungs stronger. 2. It is more effective at promoting weight loss than strength training alone (i.e., exercise for muscular endurance and strength).

For the average person who needs to lose 50 or more pounds, it can be difficult to get started in a fitness routine. When you're used to getting little or no exercise, it's difficult to get motivated to join a gym or even take a daily walk around the block. It's no big secret that as we get heavier, we find so many other things that need doing besides moving our bodies. We're too busy with our jobs, hobbies and family to devote any time to our own physical well-being.

What I like about yoga is that it doesn't have to be strenuous and, as I stated above, it's accessible for even the most sedentary among us.

Now here's where yoga provides a hidden benefit to weight loss. By going to yoga just once a week, you are *building a new habit!* You will quickly realize that you really *can* devote an hour to some form of physical activity. You will also find that you feel amazing in body and spirit after a yoga class. Before long, you will find yourself going to yoga classes perhaps twice a week. Then it's a very easy thing to add a more vigorous and aerobic form of exercise to your weekly activities! This is how my own weight loss journey began. I ended up losing 60 pounds. And it started with yoga.[10]

Trust me, you can't expect to wake up one morning and find yourself with a new habit of working out, lifting weights and running on a treadmill 5 days a week. It takes time to build a new habit of physical activity. Yoga is an easy and fun way to start building those new habits. I think of yoga as the "gateway" to the harder stuff!

Yoga quickly builds your confidence in your ability to move your body. In my years of teaching yoga I have found that everyone enjoys some form of mastery by their third class! It's amazing how quickly they improve in each pose, especially balance poses like tree and poses that require strength. In as little as a week and a half, most people go from holding a warrior pose for 5 seconds to holding it for 30 seconds. It's great to feel like you are actually good at something!

Give yourself a month or two of attending yoga classes once or twice a week and then decide whether you want to add a more aerobic activity to your schedule. Perhaps you would like to start walking with a friend on a regular basis. Maybe you would like to try jogging, swimming, biking or using an elliptical machine. Be patient with yourself. Only a month or two of yoga is needed to develop that new habit of devoting time to the betterment of your physical well-being.

Try Power Yoga to Lose Weight Faster and Improve Cardiovascular Fitness

Aerobic exercise promotes faster weight loss than strength training.[11] Power yoga provides a great aerobic workout and will help you lose weight faster than a beginner yoga class or a Hatha yoga class.

Power yoga may be too much of a challenge at first. But after a month of regular yoga, the previously sedentary person might like to give it a try. If not, then a regular program of walking, biking, running or swimming might be more suitable.

Yoga Helps You Cope With Stress

Losing weight is more about changing bad habits than about counting calories. When you change your habits of emotional eating, eating calorically dense foods and remaining sedentary, you can't help but lose weight. So how do we stop eating all the sweets and chips that are making us fat? Let's start by dealing with stress.

"A number of studies have shown that yoga can help reduce stress and anxiety. It can also enhance your mood and overall sense of well-being."[12] Yoga provides a powerful connection between mind and body and has been shown to have a significant and measurable effect on the part of our nervous system that deals with stress.[13]

Yoga's emphasis on breathing and the mind-body-spirit connection also yields strong emotional benefits. People who practice yoga frequently report that they sleep better and feel less stressed.

In general, you need to reduce your caloric intake by 3500 calories in order to lose one pound.[14] You can lose a pound a week simply by reducing your calories by 500 per day.

So, how many calories is a binge worth to you? What is a fast food meal worth? Five hundred calories? A thousand? If you can trade in your stress for a weekly yoga class and miss one binge a week, what do you think might happen? Get real and honest about your binging and overeating and portion sizes. Do the math. Who knows? You might be able to lose half a pound or even a pound a week if you can get your stress eating under control!

When You Sleep Better, You Eat Less

A study released in April, 2012 found that disrupted sleep can cause you to gain 12 pounds a year. According to sleep research done at Brigham and Women's Hospital in Boston, insufficient sleep lowers your metabolism, causes spikes in your blood sugar levels and increases your risk of diabetes.[15]   If you sleep better at night, you'll have more energy during the day and you'll be able to accomplish more.

How to Improve Your Sleep
To get a better night's rest, begin with turning off your cell phone ringer and don't eat at night. Avoid caffeine after 2 p.m. It's a good idea to sleep in a cool, dark, quiet room. If you have a

dog or cat that wakes you up in the middle of the night, perhaps she should have her own pet bed. If the problem is external noises waking you up, get an air purifier or a fan to create white noise to drown out street sounds. Perhaps you're waking up at night because your sinuses are stuffy. Maybe difficulty breathing causes you to snore and disrupts your sleep. An air purifier will help cut down on allergens. Also, Breathe Right strips will keep your sinuses open, thereby allowing you to breathe comfortably and avoid snoring. Avoid alcohol because it can cause your sinuses to swell.

If you are often tired during the day and need a nap or if your partner tells you that you snore, you may have sleep apnea. Sleep apnea is a condition where you stop breathing for a few seconds at night. It can make you snore and prevent sound sleeping. A sleep study might be warranted to see if that's a problem for you. Sleep apnea can cause serious problems and at the very least, it can make you fat.

There are many other reasons we can't sleep at night. Stress from having too much on our minds, worry and restlessness make it hard to fall asleep and stay asleep.   This is where yoga can help.

How to Improve Your Sleep with Yoga

There are many yoga routines and poses that may help you sleep at night. A gentle yoga practice can be done shortly before going to bed. The practice does not have to take an hour like a normal yoga class. In fact, you can do a few poses before going to bed, spending anywhere from 5 to 45 minutes doing so.

In a study done at **Duke University**, seven weeks of yoga was shown to improve sleep quality and to reduce the need for sleep aids in 39 adults who were experiencing insomnia while undergoing chemotherapy. Individuals who did not take the yoga sessions (control group) showed no improvement in sleep.[16]

In another study at Harvard Medical School in Boston, researchers taught 20 study participants yoga breathing, meditation and mantra. (These techniques are discussed in detail below.) The researchers found that the participants had significantly improved sleep quality at the end of treatment with yoga training compared with before the yoga training began.[17]

Pranayama Yogic Breathing Can Help You Fall Asleep

What is pranayama? Pranayama is the practice of intentional breathing that is done while practicing yoga poses. It is also done during meditation. If you have difficulty falling asleep, or if you awaken in the middle of the night and want to get back to sleep, try a calming pranayama.

My favorite calming pranayama is the **progression breath**. When I have trouble falling asleep, I inhale for the count of 4, then exhale for the count of 8. If you like, you can retain the breath for a moment after the inhalation. If you have high blood pressure, glaucoma, are pregnant or feel uncomfortable with holding the breath, please do not practice breath retention. So that's it. Inhale 4, exhale 8. Use any count that you like as long as the exhalation is twice as long as the inhalation. Chances are you'll be asleep within 3 or 4 rounds. If you wake up in the middle of the night, use the progression breath to get back to sleep.

This calming breath can also be used whenever you are upset and need to collect yourself.

Several other yogic breathing exercises (pranayama) that can be used to calm the mind or to energize the body are described below.

Meditation for Weight Loss

Stress drives a lot of us to overeat. Meditation can help you lose weight by helping you to manage your stress. It's very common to gain weight when we are under stress because most of us often use food to help us cope and to calm us. Meditation can help bring your attention to your thoughts and actions surrounding food and emotions. By using meditation in conjunction with intentionally changing your habits you will find it easier to drop those pounds.

What is meditation and how do you do it?
There are zillions of ways to meditate. Meditation can be done while sitting, standing or walking. You can meditate with your eyes open or closed. You can focus on your breath or on a word or phrase (mantra) or on an object such as a stone, candle or flower.

When you meditate your mind will wander. This is known as the "monkey mind." Our minds are like little monkeys swinging from one thought branch to another. With meditation and focusing on our breath or on a mantra or both, we calm that little monkey down. It's important to not feel like we have failed when stray thoughts pass by. We don't judge them. We simply bring our awareness back to our breath or any other focus of concentration. The idea is to be a witness to our thoughts. We quiet the mind and let go of the little stories we tell ourselves.

For the sake of simplicity, I will address only one method of meditation here.

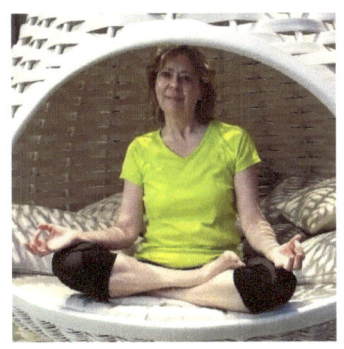 **Your mind is like the ocean.** When the waters are turbulent, you can't see your hand in front of your face. But when the surface is calm and smooth like glass, you can see the treasures that lie beneath.

1. Sit straight in a comfortable, quiet place. You can sit cross-legged on the floor or on a cushion or sit comfortably on a chair. (It's best to meditate sitting up rather than lying down so that you don't fall asleep.)
2. Close your eyes and relax.
3. Your hands might be on your knees. You might choose to use one of the hand gestures (mudras) described below.
4. Pay attention to your slow and natural breathing.
5. In your mind, you can recite this mantra, "I accept. I allow." Inhale, "I accept." Exhale, "I allow." Or choose any mantra described below. You can even make up your own!
6. When distracting thoughts occur, simply notice them and gently bring your attention back to the breath and/or your mantra. Distracting thoughts are like ripples on the ocean. Let them pass you by. Accept that they are there, allow them to wash ashore.

Try to practice meditation once a day. Set a timer for 2 minutes the first time you meditate. (Surely you can stand anything for 2 minutes!)

Meditation timer apps are available for all cell phones and other devices. Find one with pleasant gongs or chimes to gently bring you out of your meditation. You can gradually work up to a 5 minute meditation or even an hour. It is up to you. There are few rules and most of the above are only suggestions.

With time, meditation will bring to you a sense of relaxation and peace. And in that peacefulness, you may find the strength to make better food choices. You may find that you can let go of stressful situations knowing that you can meditate instead of diving into a bag of cookies.

This basic method of meditation will form the basis of our chakra meditation practices below.[18] Each chakra discussion features both a meditation practice and a mudra practice.[19] The **meditation practice** is more of a formal sit-down meditation described above whereas the **mudra practice** can serve as a quickie to get you through challenging situations.

We've seen how yoga, yogic breathing (pranayama) and meditation can help us lose weight by building muscle, helping us cope with stress and getting a good night's sleep. Now let's go deeper and explore mantras, mudras and chakras!

Mantras

What is a mantra? Mantras are words or phrases that can be repeated out loud or only in the mind. Mantras are believed to have psychological and spiritual power. A mantra may or may not have a literal meaning. The spiritual value of a mantra comes when it is audible, visible or present in thought. [20]

The sound of some mantras are said to vibrate so as to impact our chakra energy centers.[21] "There are also reflex points on the roof of the mouth that send signals to the brain to trigger specific areas in the body. So by saying a mantra, you further enhance the connection between the brain and the specific chakra by stimulating these reflex points on the roof of the mouth."[22]

A well-known use of mantra is the chanting of the word "Ohm."

Mantras do not have to be in a foreign language. You can try repeating the word "one" or you may use "one-two, one-two" when you meditate. You can also make up your own affirmation mantras to help you stay focused on your intention. We will use these affirmation mantras in the mudra hand practices. Your mantra might be, "I am relaxed." As you inhale, think, "I am." As you exhale, think, "relaxed." It's that easy. "I am....relaaaaaxed." Many other affirmation mantras are offered in this book.

Mudra Hand Gestures

If you are new to yoga, you may not be aware of the more esoteric, spiritual aspects of yoga. I call this "the woo-woo stuff." Much of the woo-woo stuff is based on thousands of years of yogic and Hindu scripture, tradition and culture. Whether you believe in the metaphysical aspects of these spiritual practices or not, you must admit that ritual has a purpose in every culture. By engaging in these chakra, mantra or mudra rituals, we bring our intention into focus. In this book, our intentions concern building healthy eating patterns and exercise habits. As we do so, we devote time, energy and concentration to working out the things that challenge us in life. So, you don't have to be a Hindu, you don't need to live in a cave on a mountain and you don't have to "believe in" anything to benefit from these lovely rituals. Keep an open mind and enjoy the process!

What is a mudra? A mudra (pronounced moo-drah) is a hand gesture or pose that helps us to cultivate a state of mind. Specific hand positions are thought to lock in energy patterns via reflex points on the fingers which correspond to different parts of the body, not unlike acupressure and acupuncture. Activating these points is said to cause a shift in the chakra energy system. According to my teacher, Tammy Zee, "mudras can be practiced anywhere and anytime. When we practice mudras it is like meditation; we merge breath, visualization, affirmations, purpose, and intention. Mudras can be practiced every day and as much as you want."

Some mudras act like affirmations or reminders of our intentions. For example, a mudra might represent courage, compassion or wisdom. Mudras are held during meditation, during some yoga poses or during yogic breathing exercises (pranayama).[23] But mudras in conjunction with affirmations are also held as a mudra practice in their own right.

Mudras show us that that which we seek is already within us. They help us to translate our intentions into skillful action.[24] Mudras bring our energy into focus on the issues with which we struggle. The practice of mudra brings self-awareness, self-control and self-realization.

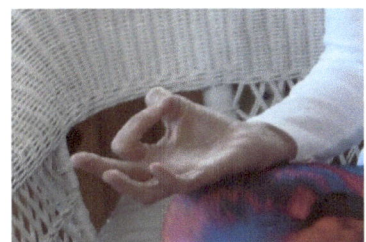 Probably the most well-known mudra, frequently seen in Indian art, is the **gyan mudra** (pictured) where the thumb and the index finger touch. This mudra signifies knowledge and wisdom and draws our focus to the unified nature of human consciousness.[25] It also reminds you to believe in yourself.

Let's try it out! To practice this mudra, sit comfortably on a chair or cross legged on a cushion. Place your hands on your knees, palms up, thumbs to index fingers. Bring your attention to your breath as it goes in and out of your body.

> I *know* that I can do this, that I *can* lose weight. I *can* control what and how much I eat. I have faith in myself that I can maintain an exercise or yoga routine once a week. My mantra now and as I go through my day is, "I believe in myself. Nothing gets in my way."

You may use any mantra phrase of your choosing to help you focus. Continue to sit quietly and breathe for 30 seconds. There! Was that so hard?

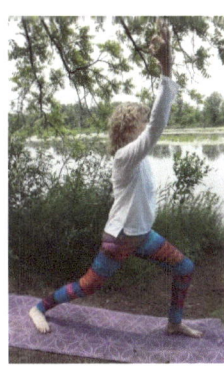 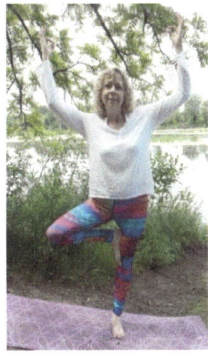 Many mudras can easily be practiced while doing Hatha yoga. It is fun and graceful to practice gyan mudra while doing Warrior

1 (left) or Warrior 2 and while doing Tree pose (right). (See previous page.)

Another mudra that can help you in your weight loss journey is Thunderbolt Mudra. The **thunderbolt mudra** (pictured) represents powerfully focused energy. Use this mudra to remove self-doubt. To practice this mudra, sit comfortably and 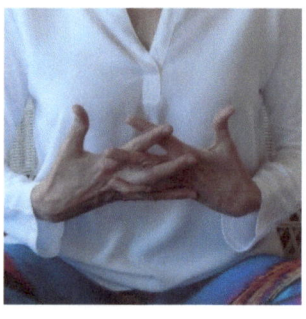 loosely interlace your fingers, held near your heart. Know that you are strong and can overcome all obstacles. You may use any mantra of your choosing to help you focus, such as "I can overcome this. I am strong!" Continue to sit quietly and breathe for 30 seconds.

In this book you will see two mudras that relate to each chakra. The first mudra will be part of your "**Chakra Meditation Practice**." This mudra is meant to help *balance the chakra* to which it resonates.

The second mudra in each chakra chapter will be a hand gesture held briefly *to bring your health and weight loss intentions into focus*. A mantra phrase is given in each "**Mudra Practice**" section. If you like, you may spend more than the suggested time with this mudra, settling down to meditate. Or simply use the mudra gesture and recite the affirmation whenever you feel the need to gather your strength and your resolve to stay strong.

It is recommended that you practice a mudra for 10 breaths. You may also work up to 11 minutes if you like. And, of course, it's fine to just hold a mudra briefly to set your intention in the moment. For example, when I find myself in a challenging situation like reaching for a bag of Ruffles in the grocery store, I stop myself long enough to practice thunderbolt mudra. To anyone passing me by, it just looks like I'm thinking about what to make for dinner tonight. The hand gesture isn't all that out of place so I don't feel self-conscious.

Chakras

What are chakras? Well, this is where it gets really *really* "woo-woo" and fun!

In Sanskrit, "chakra" (pronounced with a hard "ch" as in "chill") means "wheel." Energy is thought to radiate through the body rising from the Root Chakra at the base of the spine and pelvic floor up through the Crown Chakra at the top of the head. This path of energy is thought of as a tube called sushumna and correlates with the spine and central nervous system. Energy also radiates in a downward direction from the Crown Chakra to the Root Chakra. These two channels of energy meet at 7 main points where it is thought that they create a vortex and spin in a clockwise or counter-clockwise direction, depending on the individual.[26] When any one of these wheels of energy is blocked or out of balance, it may spin in its opposite direction or the energy may radiate outward. A chakra blockage may occur due to illness, injury or stress. Every chakra, when out of balance, can cause weight gain or prevent weight loss. When the chakras are in balance, energy moves freely, creating health, vitality, harmony and emotional well-being. You can unblock your chakras with various methods such as meditation, mudra practice, yoga, pranayama or, (are you ready for this?), the use of healing crystals and essential oils.[27]

Each of the seven main chakras relates to a part of the body and glandular system, and to an emotional or spiritual state. In fact, each chakra correlates to groupings of nerves that come off of the spine. For the purpose of this book, I will address each chakra only as it may help us in weight loss.

Root Chakra

The **Root Chakra** is often considered as the **first chakra**, and resides at the base of the spine.[28] Known as the **Muladhara Chakra**, it represents your foundation and stability. It is here that the downward current brings your ideas into reality. It is associated with your ability to feel safe and secure. The Root Chakra is about your survival which includes food, shelter, work, home, money and health. Emotionally it connects you to your self-esteem and trust of others. When this chakra is out of balance you may suffer from food addictions, a sense of scarcity, depression and low self-esteem.

When this chakra is in balance, you may feel a sense of safety and fulfillment and a feeling of belonging and fitting in.

To align your Root Chakra, you can take a yoga class, practice meditation or practice a weight loss mudra described below. Other ways to bring your chakra into balance are to wear a color that resonates with this chakra, use essential oils or

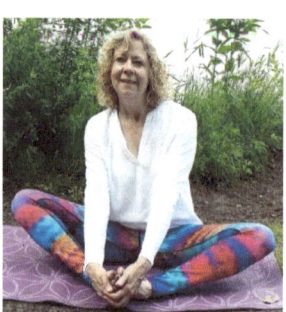

wear gemstones that relate to the Root Chakra.

Yoga Practice

When doing **yoga**, bring your attention to the Root Chakra when doing Cobbler Bound Angle Pose (pictured) or

Mountain Pose (standing tall). These poses will help to connect you to the earth. For a list of yoga poses targeting each chakra, please see Appendix A. For a copy of this list, go to www.ColorMyYoga.com and click on the Downloads tab.

Meditation Practice

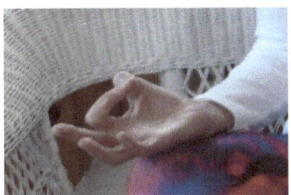

Sit comfortably, close your eyes, relax, and breathe slowly and naturally. While meditating, (as described in the meditation chapter), use the **gyan mudra** (pictured). Simply touch your thumbs to your index fingers. Begin with 3 to 5 rounds of the 4 to 8 breath (described in the pranayama chapter), inhaling for a count of 4 and exhaling for a count of 8. Press the fingertips harder during exhalation if you want a calming effect. Visualize the color red as you meditate.

To bring this chakra into balance chant the mantra that resonates with the Muladhara Chakra, "lam." Chant out loud "L-A-A-A-A-M" 3 to 5 times before settling in to your meditation. Notice the vibration as you chant! When distracting thoughts come into your mind, recognize that they are there and let them go. Meditate as long as you like, from 2 to 45 minutes.

Mudra Practice

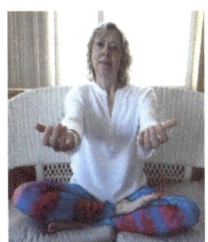

The weight loss mudra (pictured) is practiced by extending your arms in front of you, palms ups with your hands slightly cupped. Move your hands back toward your sides and then return them into the reaching out position, maintaining a 3 inch separation. Do this mudra several times, feeling the energy building up as the hands come back toward each other each time. I do this mudra in my car before going into a restaurant or before leaving my house for a party.[29]

A **mantra** that might be helpful is, "I am ready to release old habits that no longer serve me."[30] Reciting your mantra silently while walking or gardening will make you feel more connected to the earth.

Whenever you need it, practice your mudra quickly and recite your affirmation. Practicing your mudra and self-affirming mantras whenever you are feeling powerless over your food choices will help you to summon your inner strength to live a healthier life.

Stones, Colors, Oils and Foods

The **colors** connected to the root chakra are red and yellow.[31] For a list of colors that resonate with each chakra, see Appendix B. Wearing garnet jewelry or a piece of red or yellow clothing might help if you feel that your Root Chakra is out of balance. If you would like to try **essential oils**, bergamot is nice to wear. It can also be used in a diffuser.[32] For a list of chakras and their associated essential oils, see Appendix C. For a copy of these lists, go to www.ColorMyYoga.com and click on the Downloads tab.

The **food** associated with the Root Chakra is any protein. Eating protein is an excellent choice for your first meal of the day. Choosing protein and vegetables while limiting high-glycemic index carbohydrates like white bread and potatoes can help you reduce cravings and control the urge to overeat later.[33]

Because the color of this chakra is red, choosing red foods like tomatoes and red bell peppers can aid in your weight loss program. You might choose marinara sauce over a cream sauce when you go out for pasta. Red bell peppers are nature's candy. They are naturally sweet and are the perfect choice for dipping in hummus. Apples and strawberries are good choices to satisfy your sweet tooth. If your refrigerator is kept stocked with washed and ready-to-go fruit you will always have a quick and healthy snack in an "emergency."

A recipe for homemade hummus is available on www.ColorMyYoga.com by clicking on the Recipes tab. Look for other high protein recipes like deviled eggs or herb crusted salmon.

Sacral Chakra

The second chakra is the Sacral Chakra also known as Svadhistana Chakra. It is located in the lower abdomen, lower back and sex organs.

This chakra relates to your ability to be in touch with your **emotions** and to being able to identify when you are upset about something and deal with it. Too often, we may medicate our free floating feelings of hurt, embarrassment, stress, anger, guilt, shame, low self-worth and overwhelm with a pint of ice cream. We are out of touch with our feelings and so we turn to junk food to cope. Our comfort food choice is never carrots and spinach!

The Sacral Chakra is involved in how you handle relationships. When this chakra is out of balance, it affects your sexuality, your ability to connect with others and your ability to experience pleasure. Common characteristics of an unbalanced Sacral Chakra are emotional numbness, addiction to sugar, fear of change, boredom and lack of passion and excitement.

If you are overweight and feel that this chakra might be out of balance, it will come as no surprise that the sense connected to the Svadhistana Chakra is the sense of taste! Let me show you how you can turn your sense of taste into your new super power!

To feed your body good and nutritious food, start by paying attention to ingredient labels. Foods made with the same ingredients you find in your kitchen are better than those with a long list of hard-to-pronounce additives. Try to avoid added fats and sugars. If possible, cook your meals from scratch.

Notice the taste difference between natural, un-messed-with food and overly processed packaged food that is full of chemicals. The next time you have boxed macaroni and cheese ask yourself if it really tastes like cheese. Question your cappuccino. Cappuccinos at a gas station list sugar as the first ingredient followed by a list of chemicals like mono and di-glycerides and something called DATEM. Most bottled salad dressings are so full of fillers and emulsifiers that they don't come close to tasting like the real thing.[34] I've even seen prime rib in a grocery store deli case that contained 41 ingredients, most of which were chemicals! Why?

Using your new super power, have fun doing some taste comparisons. Try Newman's salad dressing and compare it to one that contains mono and di-glycerides to see the difference. Compare self-serve gas station cappuccino to a real cappuccino at a café. There's that glyceride flavor again! Using your new taste bud super power you can learn to enjoy real food! Honor your body and give it only chemical-free, nourishing, tasty and *real* food.

Meditation Practice

The belly breath is a helpful **pranayama** for meditation when working on the Sacral Chakra. To begin **meditation**, hold one hand on your belly and one on your chest and breathe fully and deeply to allow your lower lungs to inflate, causing your belly to expand. Inhale slowly and deeply 3 to 5 times while focusing on your Sacral Chakra and your chakra color, orange or white.

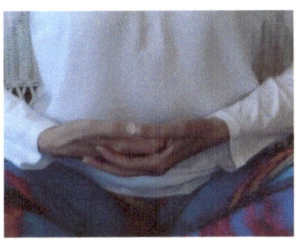

To unblock the Sacral Chakra, the Mudra that we use while meditating is the dhyana mudra (pictured) with left hand in the lap, right hand on top of left, palms up. The mantra that assists in bringing this chakra into balance is "vam". Chant out loud "V-A-A-A-A-M" 3 times. Let the sound really vibrate and resonate. Then relax and meditate.

Mudra Practice

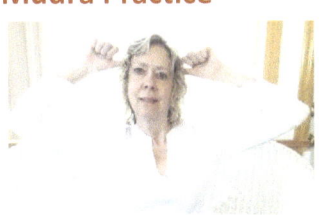

The **mudra for overcoming addictive habits** (pictured) should be practiced three times a day for three minutes for 30 days. Sit calmly with your back straight. Make a fist with each hand and press the thumbs firmly to the temples. Clench your jaws, left jaw, right jaw, alternating back and forth, feeling the pressure under each thumb.[35] Use this mudra before you go grocery shopping. Set your intention to purchase only healthy foods. Refuse to give in to your food addictions. Stay out of the ice cream aisle and don't go near the snack aisle! If you don't buy it, you can't eat it. Use this handy mudra whenever the urge arises to cruise the cupboards for carbs.

The **sat-nam mantra** moves energy up to the Heart Chakra to release **addiction**. "Sat" rhymes with "what," and means "truth" while "nam," pronounced na-am, means "embodied essence."[36] Recite, chant or think your mantra, "sat nam," several times after your mudra practice. You can recite it silently whenever you are faced with one of your cravings.

Yoga Practice

Yoga poses that benefit and balance the Sacral Chakra are camel (pictured), lotus and forward fold. And here's a bonus. A good exercise for bringing the Sacral Chakra back into balance is to have sex! ☺

Stones, Colors, Oils and Foods

Jasmine essential oil brings balance to the Sacral Chakra. Use it in your bath or on your skin. You can also add it to a spray bottle filled with water to spritz in the air whenever you want to freshen up your house. A jasmine scented candle would be a nice focal point for meditation.

If you would like to wear gemstones to help align the Svadhistana Chakra, choose moonstone, orange tourmaline or tiger eye. Wear a piece of clothing with one of your Sacral Chakra colors, orange or white.

Food choices to promote and maintain this chakra are water and tea. You may also choose a water-based orange food like oranges and tangerines. This would rule out cheese puffs if you're trying to eat orange colors! Peeled oranges will keep in the refrigerator for several days. Preparing them ahead of time makes it easier to make this healthy choice when you are cruising the kitchen for a snack. Orange bell peppers, like the red peppers, are naturally sweet and work great as a dip delivery system! For a low calorie yummy chip dip recipe, visit www.ColorMyYoga.com and click on the Recipes tab. The dip is made with nonfat Greek yogurt in place of sour cream. It truly tastes as good as sour cream dip!

Is anything yummier than papaya? Go ahead and enjoy papaya chunks as-is or added to a vegetable salad or fruit salad. Splurge with a mango. Both are sweet and filled with nutrients, fiber and naturally occurring sugars. Carrots and yams make excellent side dishes. And sweet potato fries are easy to make in the toaster oven. The sweet potato fries recipe is available on the website too.

Because the **element** of water is integral to the Sacral Chakra, a bubble bath is also beneficial. Children's bath colors may be added to the water. A red tablet and a yellow tablet make orange.[37] Essential oils may be added to the bath, but avoid citrus oils which can be irritating to the skin.

Solar Plexus Chakra

The **Solar Plexus Chakra** or **Manipura** Chakra is the seat of your will and the focus of your metabolism and digestion. Willpower and metabolism; isn't that what weight loss is all about? Energy and intention must be in balance with each other. With good intentions and no energy to put into your intention, your will is weakened. If you don't pay attention to the food (energy) you put in your body, your metabolism suffers. The solar plexus is your power center and is the area of your assertiveness, intuition and inner drive.

Signs that your Third Chakra is out of sync are eating disorders, digestion problems, low energy, low self-esteem and weak willpower. But when your Manipura Chakra is balanced and healthy, you have great self-control, confidence and energy. The word "manipura" means "filled with gems." Bringing the Solar Plexus Chakra back into balance will reveal your inner gems of self-control, confidence and energy. You can more easily align your intentions with your actions.

You can resist peer pressure when you have a stronger sense of self. By bringing your Solar Plexus Chakra into balance, You can feel stronger and more able to resist your family's insistence on a second piece of birthday cake. You can resist the peer pressure from your friends to split a dessert when you are already full. You can resist the peer pressure to feel shamed into ordering a salad when what you really need is protein. With a balanced and healthy Solar Plexus Chakra, you can stop seeking the approval of others. But when you let go of your personal power, others can easily shame you into actions that fulfill *their* needs rather than your own.

"Have another piece of pie. One more won't hurt." "No thanks. I'm working on my Solar Plexus Chakra today!" That'll stop them in their tracks!

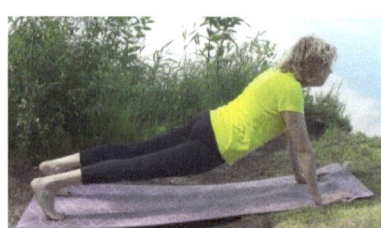

Yoga Practice
Plank pose (pictured) is a yoga pose as well as an exercise to increase

abdominal strength. To do this exercise, come into a push-up position resting on your hands with elbows locked and straight and your torso parallel to the floor. You can also perform plank pose resting on your elbows. The elbow position works your abs even more than the hand position, but it is easier on the wrists. If this pose is too difficult, you may practice it with your hands on the 4th or 5th step of a stairway. Drop down a step as you build strength. In plank pose, modified or not, keep your torso straight and hold for 5 to 60 seconds. Your goal when you are first starting out is to hold the pose for a total of 60 seconds, whether it's 60 all at once or 5 seconds at a time. When you eventually master a 60 second hold without resting, then begin working toward doing 3 sets of 60 second holds. This pose builds your abdominal muscles while helping to balance the Sacral Chakra. Use this pose to tap into your new willpower!

Meditation practice

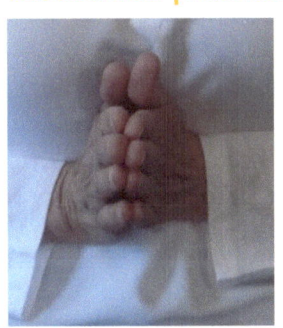

When you wish to balance your Solar Plexus Chakra, take a couple of minutes in the morning to meditate with the **anjali mudra** (pictured), a gesture of meditation and of reverence. In anjali mudra, the hands are in prayer position. You hold the heels of your hands between the heart and the stomach with finger tips pointing forward. "Ram" is the **mantra** to open the Manipura Chakra. Chant this mantra out loud, letting your voice resonate "R-A-A-A-A-M."[38] Visualize the color yellow as you meditate.

Two mudras are offered here, one for stoking your metabolism and the other to help you persevere in the face of temptations.

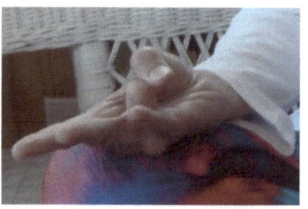

Surya Ravi Mudra (pictured) helps to heat the body and raise the metabolism. Thus, it is an excellent posture for those who want to lose weight. Surya is the Sanskrit word for the Sun and the Surya Mudra is so called because it increases the element of fire in the body. Bend the ring finger of each hand so that its tip touches the mound of your thumb. Press down on your ring finger with your thumb. Ensure that the other fingers are spread out straight. As you inhale, apply more pressure to the fingertips to develop determination and to energize your metabolism.

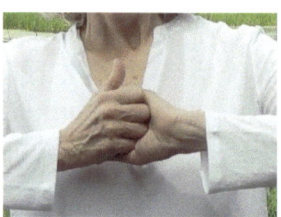

Ganesha Mudra (pictured) is named for the elephant god, Ganesha. Nothing stands in the way of an elephant and Ganesha is seen as the god of success. This mudra is recommended to help remove all obstacles from your path, lift your spirits and give you the will to persevere when you are feeling down. Bring both hands in front of your chest with your elbows bent. Position the left hand with the palm facing outwards in such a way that your thumb is on the bottom and your little finger is on top. Form a claw by bending the four fingers of your left hand and clasp them with the four fingers of your right hand. In this position, your right palm should be facing towards your chest. Inhale deeply. On the exhale, try to pull both arms apart while keeping all eight fingers locked. Feel the stretch along your shoulders and chest. Inhale once more and relax your arms while maintaining the Ganesha Mudra lock. Repeat this process six times. Interchange your hands, with your right palm facing outwards and the left palm facing inwards and repeat this process.

This mudra comes in handy when you want to go to a spin class (success) but your best friend insists that you skip your workout and go out for breakfast (obstacle). This mudra is also useful when you are on your way into a restaurant and worried about overdoing it (obstacle). It will do wonders for your ability to remain steadfast and strong in your quest to regain your health (success).

The following affirming mantra is part of your mudra practice. "I am powerful, determined and strong enough to follow through with my goals."

Stones, Colors, Oils and Foods
An essential oil that serves the Solar Plexus Chakra is peppermint. The colors yellow and red are associated with the Solar Plexus Chakra.

Wearing citrine, jasper or topaz gemstones might help focus your willpower to choose physical activity over sitting on the couch and nutrient dense foods over calorie dense foods. Wearing yellow or red clothing will remind you to stay strong and focused while you build new healthier habits and strengthen your willpower.

Eating yellow vegetables and fruits is said to support the Solar Plexus Chakra as well. (No, boxed mac 'n cheese doesn't count!) Try adding a wedge of lemon to sparkling water to wean yourself off of sugary sodas and artificially sweetened sodas. Enjoy a half grapefruit sprinkled with one or two teaspoons of real sugar for breakfast. Add bananas to a fruit smoothie for a yummy and nutritious breakfast or mid-afternoon meal. For a really easy smoothie recipe, visit www.ColorMyYoga.com and click on the Recipes tab.

Heart Chakra

The Heart Chakra is located at the center of the chest. This chakra, the **Anahata** Chakra, is thought to control the heart and lungs.

The Sanskrit word "anahata" means "unhurt". "To open the heart is to treat others (as well as things), with honor and respect and to refrain from causing unnecessary harm. An open heart feels **compassion** and **empathy** for both self and others." [39] The Heart Chakra is thought of as the balancing point between the three lower physical chakras and the three higher spiritual chakras.[40]

When your Heart Chakra is out of balance, you may have feelings of depression, abandonment, isolation, and loneliness; all of which seem like a good excuse to dive into a pint of Haggen-daaz. You may lack compassion for yourself, coming down hard on yourself when you give into a binge. The fact that your Heart Chakra is in disrepair may also be evident when anger and resentment are eating at you.

But when this chakra is in balance, you may feel more willing to share and give of yourself. You can enjoy a sense of hope, self-acceptance and health. You can also engage in relationships with others in a more positive way.

Self-compassion is necessary to losing weight and maintaining a healthy diet. It is so easy to give up on yourself after you overeat. You may feel like you will never be able to stick to a diet or lose weight. Bashing yourself over a slip-up isn't going to accomplish anything. In fact, it's counter-productive. "Study after study shows that self-criticism [is] consistently associated with less motivation and worse self-control...Self-compassion - being supportive and kind to yourself, especially in the face of stress and failure - is associated with more motivation and better self-control."[41]

"A healthy heart chakra has the power to transform love into healing energy. Because love is the most nourishing energy, the heart chakra has the ability to balance all the other chakras through its expression of love."[42] With a healthy balanced Heart Chakra, you can give yourself the love and compassion that you deserve as you continue on your path to better health.

Yoga Practice

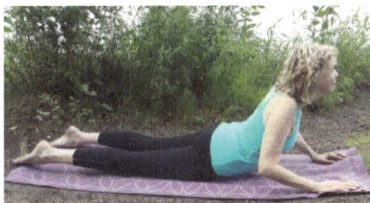

As part of your yoga practice and to aid in bringing your Heart Chakra back into balance, focus on chest opening poses like camel or cobra (pictured).

Meditation practice

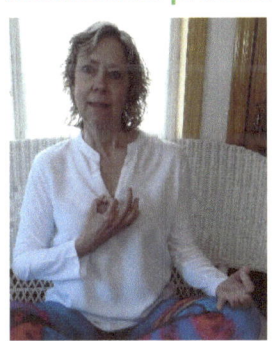

In seeking self-compassion, you need to balance your Heart Chakra with meditation. Begin your Heart Chakra meditation, with thumbs to index fingers in gyan **mudra** (pictured). Place the "O" formed by the fingers of the right hand to your heart. The left hand in gyan mudra rests on your left knee. Chant the Heart Chakra mantra "yam," ("Y-A-A-A-M") out loud three to five times. Breathe slowly and relax. As you exhale, press your fingers together harder to increase the calming effect. Visualize the color green as you meditate.

After your mantra, you may practice the alternate nostril pranayama known as nadi shodhana. This is a calming breath that helps with stress and anxiety. Essentially, you inhale through the right side and exhale through the left, then inhale left and exhale right. If you do not have high blood pressure, glaucoma or are pregnant you may hold your breath momentarily after an inhale. To do nadi shodhana, use your right thumb to press your right nostril. Place the ring and middle fingers (same hand) against the left nostril. Proceed as follows: press the left nostril – inhale through the right side – press the right – exhale through the left. Then, inhale left, press left, exhale right. Repeat: inhale right, press, exhale left, inhale left, press, exhale right. In other words, you inhale on one side, press that side and then exhale that breath through the other side and inhale on that side before switching. It's really not as complicated as it sounds. Do 5 to 10 rounds, paying attention to your own comfort level. Then settle into a few minutes of meditation.

Mudra Practice

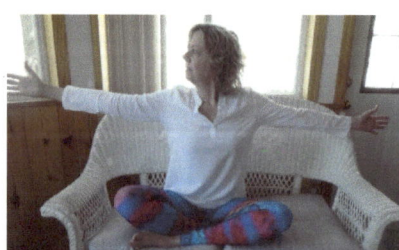

The **mudra for compassion** (pictured) helps you to count your blessings and feel compassion for yourself and others. To do compassion mudra, sit with your arms spread wide. Concentrate on your heart center while turning your head side to side. Turn to the right and back to center 4 times and then to the left and back to center 4 times. Experience compassion for yourself and everyone in your life.[43]

Your mantra or affirmation might be, "I forgive myself for a slip-up. Tomorrow is a new day." Another affirmation is one of gratitude. "I am grateful for the blessings in my life, for my healthy body and for the abundance of healthy and nutritious food." Gratitude for what we have and forgiveness for things that have gone wrong invite our heart to open. Practice and meditate on forgiving yourself, opening your heart to those around you and feeling compassion toward yourself. You're only human. Use your forgiveness and gratitude mantras whenever you notice you are criticizing yourself. The regular practice of compassion mudra will help you to feel forgiveness for not being perfect. Practicing your abundance mantra will help you feel gratitude for all that you are and appreciation for all that you have.

Stones, Colors, Oils and Foods

To keep you focused on your intention to open your heart and practice self-compassion, you might choose rose as your essential oil. This oil is said to have properties that balance the Heart Chakra. Try a little mixed with lotion for dry hands, knees and feet or add a few drops to your bath. For other essential oils, see Appendix C.

The **color** of the Heart Chakra is considered to be green or smoke. To aid in bringing the Heart Chakra into alignment, it is suggested that you add more green foods to your diet. No, not green M&M's and Mountain Dew! ☺ Choose salads and other nutrient dense green foods like avocados, chives, herbs, asparagus, spinach, kale, collard greens and broccoli. Keep a bowl of seedless green grapes handy for a late afternoon snack when sugar cravings are at their worst. For a salad recipe, visit www.ColorMyYoga.com and click on the Recipes tab.

Wearing a green garment or scarf or perhaps something made with filmy sheer fabric can remind you of your quest for self-compassion. Wear emerald, rose quartz or ruby stones to remind you to practice kindness to yourself. In keeping your attention centered on compassion, pledge to do no harm to your own spirit or that of others. One way to avoid self-harm is to refrain from punishing your body with poor food choices.

Throat Chakra

The Throat Chakra, known as Vishuddha (pronounced vish-ood-dah), is located in the throat and governs communication, listening, speaking, creativity, self-expression and speaking one's truth. The Sanskrit word "Vishuddha" means "pure" in the sense of honesty and it relates to "right speech."

Signs that there is deficiency in this, the fifth chakra are thyroid, throat or sinus problems and swearing. (Please consult a physician if you think you may have a thyroid problem. Hypothyroid, underactive thyroid, can lead to weight gain.)

Notice the negative energy that wells up whenever you use a swear word. The throat chakra will benefit if you can find new words that are less emotionally charged to express displeasure. Try turning negative thoughts into positive ones. Problems become challenges and road blocks become opportunities.

When your Throat Chakra is out of balance, you aren't saying what needs to be said. You might find yourself swallowing your feelings rather than voicing them. You feel off balance. This can lead to binge eating as a way to take your mind off your feelings. Creative endeavors such as singing and keeping a journal will help you find your voice and bring balance to this chakra.

Yoga Practice

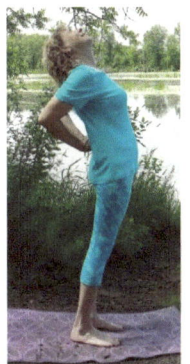

When your purpose is in opening and balancing the Vishuddha Chakra, your yoga practice can include cobra, backbends (pictured) and shoulder stand.[44]

Meditation practice

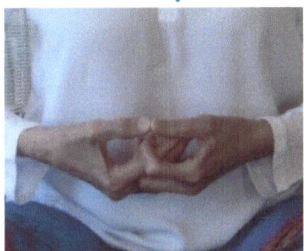

Sit in a comfortable position as described in the meditation chapter. Hands will be in the Throat Chakra mudra (pictured). This mudra is done with hands in front of the tummy, fingers interlaced and the tips of the thumbs touching each other.

"Ham" is the sound that resonates in the Throat Chakra. Chant the sound "H-A-A-A-M" out loud three times. Follow this mantra with a nice calming "three part breath." Begin by breathing into the belly then the chest and then the neck. Reverse by exhaling from the neck, then the chest then the belly. Practice just 3 or 4 rounds at the beginning of your meditation.

Mudra Practice

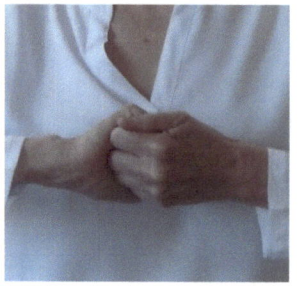

Speak your truth. When the Throat Chakra is in balance, you can speak up for yourself in a way that does not harm yourself or others. To empower your own inner voice, the vocal empowerment mudra (pictured) is recommended. This is similar to the Ganesha mudra. Bring your hands to your heart. Your right palm faces away from you, your left palm faces toward you. Clasp the fingers of one hand to the fingers of the other and bring your thumbs in to create fists.

Practice **ujjayi breath**. This **pranayama**, also called the ocean breath, requires that you restrict the glottis, making an audible "Darth Vader" sound as you exhale through the mouth. If you are alone, then make your ujjayi breath as loud as you can. Feel your power. Close your eyes, relax, inhale and exhale slowly. Collapse the belly, drawing it in as you exhale, emptying your lungs.[45] In your mind, recite this mantra, "I celebrate the beauty in my life."

You may practice this mudra and pranayama for 2 or 3 minutes as you set your intention for the day. The vocal empowerment mudra comes in handy whenever you feel you are being run over by other people. It may also be used when you need to stand up for yourself.

Stones, Colors, Oils and Foods

Set your intention today to practice right speech and thereby purify your Throat Chakra. Speak only of others as if they were in your presence. Remind yourself of your intention by wearing turquoise clothing or a filmy scarf the color of sea water. Wear jewelry that is made with aquamarine, blue opal or carnelian **gem stones**. An **essential oil** that is thought to help balance the Throat Chakra is oil of orange. For others, see Appendix C.

Blue berries and blackberries are said to help balance the Throat Chakra. Pears and peaches may also help.

Third Eye Chakra

The 6th chakra is located between and above the eyes where we perceive the third eye to be and in the pituitary gland. This chakra is called **Ajna**, the overseer. The Third Eye Chakra is related to sight and seeing, both intuitively and physically. It is connected to light, clairvoyance, intuition, intelligence, wisdom, intellect, imagination, telepathy, dreams, thinking clearly and the sixth sense. Focus on what could be rather than on what is.[46] The main issue is in trusting your inner guidance and intuition.[47]

Though the Third Eye Chakra seems at first glance to have little to do with your weight, perhaps it has everything to do with it. The word "ajna" means both to perceive and to command. When this chakra is balanced, you can think with clear **perception**. With this powerful tool, you can **command** into being that which you focus your energy upon. Whatever you would like to manifest, or bring into being in your life, you can create by visualizing it and giving it your energy. "Many of us carry negative images – about our bodies, our self-worth or about the future. These negative images also influence manifestation, sometimes quite powerfully. Whatever you focus on has a way of increasing. If you focus on negativity, you draw it toward you. If you focus on your blessings, they will multiply."[48] Balancing this chakra may help you avoid engaging in negative self-talk.

Light is the "element" connected to the Third Eye Chakra. Use light and color to heal the Ajna Chakra. Wear brightly colored clothing. Visit an art gallery. Expose yourself to natural sun light. Keep a journal or a dream journal. Appreciate pleasant coincidences, i.e., synchronicity.

Yoga Practice

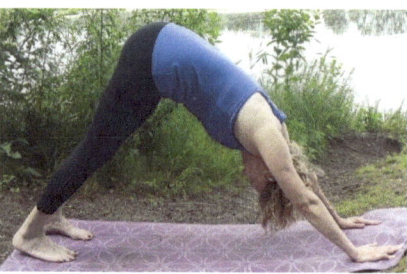

Down dog (pictured) and child pose are good poses for balancing the Ajna Chakra. Focus your mind's eye on the color indigo or clear white light while in either of these poses.

Meditation practice

To begin, place your hands in ajna **mudra** (pictured). The tips of the middle fingers touch each other and the tips of the thumbs touch each other while the second joint of the other fingers touch each other. Visualize the color indigo as you meditate.

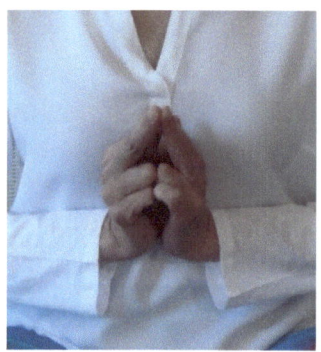

Start your meditation with one to three minutes of humming bee breath. Inhale deeply. Exhale through the mouth with the lips touching and make the sound "hmmmmmm" until your lips vibrate.[49]

The **mantra** for the third eye chakra is "Ohm." Chant out loud the word "Ohm" three times. You may do it loudly or quietly, drawing it out as long as you like. "Ohm" or "om" or "aum" is the sacred sound of the universe.

Mudra Practice

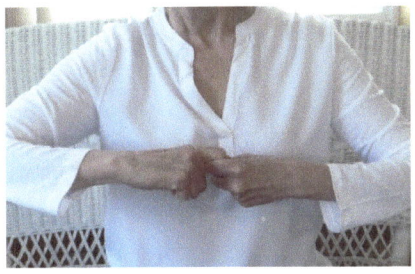

To see beyond any difficulty you are going through, you need to focus on the bigger picture. To practice the **mudra for wisdom** Tuck your thumbs under your fingers. Straighten the index fingers and hook them together. The right palm faces downward and the left palm faces your chest.[50]

The mantra is "I am united with the vibration of the infinite."[51] Chant or think this mantra 3 to 5 times. Use it whenever you find yourself engaging in negative self-talk. Practice viloma pranayama or "against the current" breath. This relaxing breath is very simple. Inhale normally, then exhale for a count of 2, hold for 2, exhale for a count of 2, hold for 2, exhale for a count of 2, hold for 2. If you have high blood pressure, glaucoma or are pregnant, you may simply skip holding the breath. Repeat this breath 3 to 5 times.

Stones, Colors, Oils and Foods

The colors associated with this chakra are indigo and snow white. To help the function of the Third Eye Chakra, you may wear amethyst, lapis lazuli or sapphire. A lovely essential oil that may help in your meditation is lavender. (For more choices, see Appendix C.) Associated foods are airy foods such as greens, green drinks, tea and bubbling mineral water. Any foods with the color violet will help balance this chakra, e.g., purple potatoes, blackberries, plums, purple grapes and figs.[52]

Crown Chakra

The 7th chakra is the Crown Chakra, or **Sahasrara** meaning thousand-fold. The Crown Chakra is pictured as a thousand petal lotus. "At the center of the lotus, your individual point of awareness connects with the overarching field of divine intelligence, knowing there is no separation. In the true meaning of the word "yoga" as union, the individual and the divine are at last linked in the common field of consciousness." [53] The lotus is the symbol of spirituality and purity.

The Sahasrara Chakra is located at the top of the head and in the pineal gland. It is considered to be the home of your **spirituality**. It contains your enlightenment, self-fulfillment and self-realization.[54] It connects you to the highest state of enlightenment. "When the Crown Chakra is balanced, it opens us to a profound awakening, like the lotus blossom when it opens. It connects us to our innate spiritual nature as well as to divine or cosmic consciousness."[55]

When the Crown Chakra is out of balance, you may experience worry and depression, chronic fatigue, addiction to mind altering drugs, anorexia and obesity. You may also suffer from exhaustion, migraines and musculoskeletal diseases.

Other problems associated with the crown chakra are issues with the sleep/wake cycle, difficulty meditating, obsession with religion, feeling disconnected from your body or others and spiritual discomfort.

When the Sahasrara Chakra is balanced, you may experience spiritual connectedness, wisdom, selflessness and open mindedness. You may experience bliss and fulfillment.

If you are overweight, a root cause might be

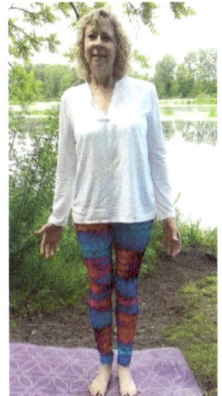

problems with the sleep cycle (discussed above) and with depression or chronic fatigue syndrome. For these of course, it is recommended that you see a physician.

Yoga Practice
Mountain pose (pictured) and downward facing dog help to align the Crown Chakra.

Meditation Practice

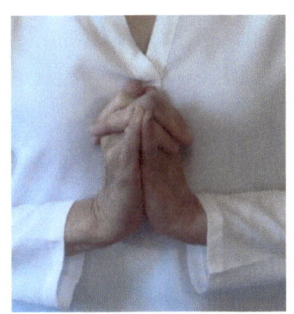

To begin your Crown Chakra meditation, place your hands in **sahasrara mudra** (pictured). Fingers are interlaced and little fingers touch each other pointing upwards. Chant out loud "ang," the sound connected to the crown chakra; "A-A-A-N-G." You may also use "aum." Visualize white light as you meditate. Breathe comfortably, slowly and naturally.

Mudra Practice

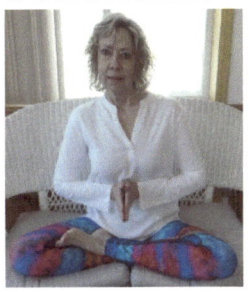

"All the answers are within you…Whenever you search consciously, you will find the answer you need." To practice the **mudra for higher consciousness** (pictured), place your hands in prayer position, heels of the hands at your solar plexus (belly button area). Right thumb sits snugly above the left thumb, palms pressed together. Breathe slowly and deeply for a minute or two.[56]

A beautiful **pranayama** is the **Breath of Balance**. Sit comfortably with an erect spine, fingertips touching the floor. Inhale lifting the arms high above your head, bringing fingertips together. Exhale while lowering the fingertips to the floor. Visualize white or violet light and universal energy flowing from the crown of your head and enveloping your body. Inhale, arms lifted, exhale, arms down. Do this for 3 minutes. Your mantra is, "I am balanced between earth and heaven."[57]

Stones, Colors, Oils and Foods

Frankincense is a nice essential oil that can bring your focus to the Sahasrara Chakra. For more choices, see Appendix C.

Gemstones that are considered associated with Crown Chakra are diamond, quartz, black opal and sunstone.

The colors connected to the Crown chakra are opal, pink, white, purple, or violet. Purple foods may help the Crown chakra. For purple and white foods, try peeled and cubed jicama added to a salad. It tastes like a cross between a potato and an apple. Sticks of jicama make excellent hummus delivery utensils! Like jicama, mushrooms are practically calorie free and add a lot of flavor and texture to other foods.

"The crown chakra is different than the rest in that it is more "spirit" than "matter." Therefore, the true food of the crown chakra is fresh air, sunlight and being out in nature.[58] To balance this chakra, move your body in nature. Go for a hike in the woods. Do yoga in a park. Soak up all the nature you can stand!

Conclusion

You now have the chakra tools to help you respond to decreased willpower. The next time you are faced with challenges to your weight loss goals, take a moment to look inward. Ask yourself what is driving you to over-indulge or to skip a workout. Which chakras do you feel are out of balance right now? Turn to the appropriate section of this book to find a mudra that will help you to stay focused on your weight loss goals. Recite a mantra to strengthen your resolve. Choose helpful essential oils and gem stones to wear. Surround yourself with the colors that remind you of your intention. Enjoy colorful foods to increase your physical energy and balance your chakra energies.

It is my wish for you that you enjoy your weight loss journey and your colorful chakra practice.

Namaste![59]

Appendix A
Yoga Poses Associated with the Chakras

For a copy of this list, go to www.ColorMyYoga.com and click on the Downloads tab.

Muladhara Root Chakra	Mountain, Cobbler and Seated Circles.
Svadhistana Sacral Chakra	Camel, Eagle, Forward Fold, Cobbler and Lotus.
Manipura Solar Plexus	Boat, Plank, Locust, Bow and Twisting Poses.
Anahata Heart Chakra	Cow Face, Alternate Nostril Breath, Cobra and Spinal Twist.
Vishuddha Throat Chakra	Lion, Cobra, Backbends, Shoulder Stand, Plow and Fish.
Ajna 3rd Eye Chakra	Child Pose, Rabbit, Down Dog, Meditation, Chanting and Inversions.
Sahasrara Crown Chakra	Head Stand, Inversions and Mountain.

Appendix B
Colors Associated with the Chakras

For a copy of this list, go to www.ColorMyYoga.com and click on the Downloads tab.

Chakra	Rainbow Colors	Vishnu-Devenanda
Root Muladhara	Red	Yellow
Sacral Svadhistana	Orange	White
Solar Plexus Manipura	Yellow	Red
Heart Anahata	Green	Smoke
Throat Vishuddha	Turquoise or Blue	Sea Water
Third Eye Ajni	Indigo	Snow White
Crown Sahasrara	Opal, Pink, White, Purple or Violet.	Vishnu-Devenanda does not assign a color to the crown chakra.

Appendix C
Essential Oils
Associated with the
Chakras

For a copy of this list, go to www.ColorMyYoga.com and click on the Downloads tab.

Chakra	Essential Oils
Root Muladhara	Bergamot, Sandalwood, Nutmeg, Cinnamon, Ginger, Myrrh and Patchouli.
Sacral Svadhistana	Sandalwood, Tangerine*, Orange*, Geranium, Texas Cedar Wood, Jasmine, Rose and Ylang-Ylang.
Solar Plexus Manipura	Myrrh, Frankincense, Balsam, Lemon*, Ginger and Peppermint.
Heart Anahata	Rose, Eucalyptus, Bergamot, Geranium, Rosemary, Peppermint, Tea Tree, Marjoram, Neroli and Pine.
Throat Vishuddha	Peppermint, Chamomile, Orange*, Rosemary, Lavender, Geranium and Coriander.
Third Eye Ajni	Lavender, Lemon*, Clary Sage, Vanilla, Bergamot and Orange.
Crown Sahasrara	Frankincense, Sandalwood, Neroli, Jasmine, Ylang Ylang and Rose.

*Citrus oils should not be added to the bath as they can be irritating to the skin.

Endnotes

[1] Why diets fail, and how weight control works | Tampa Bay Times. (n.d.). Retrieved from http://www.tampabay.com/features/fitness/why-diets-fail-and-how-weight-control-works/1079221

[2] Fit for Life: Keeping the Weight Off | Psychology Today. (n.d.). Retrieved from https://www.psychologytoday.com/articles/200201/fit-life-keeping-the-weight

[3] Dieting does not work, researchers report. (n.d.). Retrieved from http://www.physorg.com/news94906931.html

[4] Ibid.

[5] For more on this topic, see Haug, C. (2014) Rehab for Weight Loss, A Humorous Approach to Getting Skinny and Healthy [Kindle DX version]. Retrieved from Amazon.com.

[6] For more on this topic, see Haug, C. (2014) Rehab for Weight Loss, A Humorous Approach to Getting Skinny and Healthy [Kindle DX version]. Retrieved from Amazon.com.

[7] For the most part, when I use the term "yoga," I am referring to Hatha yoga and the physical practice of doing yoga poses, known as "asanas." Hatha yoga combines movement with controlled breathing or pranayama.

[8] "Yoga, Mindfulness Boost Bottom Line." Yoga Journal. N.p., 22 Mar. 2013. Web. 25 Mar. 2013.

9 The obvious exception is power yoga.

[10] For more on this topic, see Haug, C. (2014) Rehab for Weight Loss, A Humorous Approach to Getting Skinny and Healthy [Kindle DX version]. Retrieved from Amazon.com.

[11] Aerobic Exercise Trumps Resistance Training for Weight and Fat Loss - Duke Medicine. (n.d.). Retrieved from http://corporate.dukemedicine.org/news_and_publications/news_office/news/aerobic-exercise-trumps-resistance-training-for-weight-and-fat-loss.

[12] Yoga: Fight stress and find serenity - Mayo Clinic. (n.d.). Retrieved from http://www.mayoclinic.org/healthy-lifestyle/stress-management/in-depth/yoga/art-20044733.

[13] From a study in March 2013 at the University of Kansas Medical Center led by Dhanunjaya Lakkireddy, MD. The University of Kansas Hospital | Kansas City, KS. (n.d.). Retrieved from http://www.kumed.com/newsroom/news/published-study-finds-yoga-safe-effective-therapy-for-heart-patients.

[14] Actually, the 3500 calories equals a pound rule is an over-simplification of how weight loss works. The more fat you have, the more accurate the rule is. If a lean person tries to cut back 3500 calories a week, he or she will lose more muscle mass than fat. But if being lean isn't your problem right now, then stick with the 3500 calories a week rule. For further information, refer to a study done by Dr. Kevin Hall, an investigator at the National Institute of Health in Bethesda. Hall, KD., What is the required energy deficit per unit of weight loss? Int J Obesity. 2007 Epub ahead of print.

[15] Science Transactional Medicine Journal.

[16] Frontiers | Yoga on Our Minds: A Systematic Review of Yoga for Neuropsychiatric Disorders | Affective Disorders and Psychosomatic Research. (n.d.). Retrieved from http://journal.frontiersin.org/article/10.3389/fpsyt.2012.00117/abstract

[17] Yoga Helps Relieve Sleep Problems | Elaine Gavalas. (n.d.). Retrieved from http://www.huffingtonpost.com/elaine-gavalas/yoga-sleep_b_1719825.html

18 There are 7 energy points in the body known as "chakras." These energy points impact our physical and emotional wellbeing.

[19] Mudras are hand gestures or poses that help us to connect and focus on our intentions.

[20] Mantra - Wikipedia, the free encyclopedia. (n.d.). Retrieved April 25, 2015, from http://en.wikipedia.org/wiki/Mantra.

[21] Such mantras are discussed in the chapter on chakras. They are: lam (connected to the root chakra), vam (sacral chakra), ram (solar plexus), yam (heart), ham (throat), aum (third eye) and ang (crown).

[22] Find Chakra Balance Through Your Diet | The Oz Blog. (n.d.). Retrieved from http://blog.doctoroz.com/oz-experts/find-chakra-balance-through-your-diet. See also: Restore Your Health With Chakras, Pt 1 - The Secrets In Your Chakras: Seven Energy Centers | The Dr. Oz Show. (n.d.). Retrieved from http://www.doctoroz.com/episode/secrets-your-chakras-7-energy-centers?video_id=2759276191001

[23] From Hand to Heart." (2015, April). Yoga Journal, Special Meditation Issue, 92.

[24] *Ibid.*

[25] *Ibid.*, p. 93.

[26] Olivia H. Miller. (2004) The Chakra Deck. San Francisco: Chronicle Books. Miller states that the spin is clockwise. Other sources state that the spin is counter-clockwise. Some authorities maintain that the direction of spin depends on the individual. Regardless of the direction of spin, the point is that the spin will change direction when the chakra is out of balance.

[27] For further reading about the chakra system see: Olivia H. Miller. (2004) The Chakra Deck. San Francisco: Chronicle Books. Anodea Judith. (2003). Chakra Balancing. Boulder, Colorado: Sounds True. Swami Vishnu-Devananda. (1960). The Complete Illustrated Book of Yoga. New York: Three Rivers Press.

[28] The chakras are sometimes numbered from the top down. So the Root Chakra is also called the 7th chakra.

[29] Sabrina Mesko. (2013) Healing Mudras, Yoga for Your Hands (p. 62). United States: Mudra Hands Publishing.

[30] Miller, p. 6.

[31] The ancients did not assign colors to the various chakras. The color system is a modern contrivance. Judith, p. 70. Assigning colors to the chakras began in the West in the 1940's. Chakra - Wikipedia, the free

encyclopedia. (n.d.). Retrieved April 25, 2015, from http://en.wikipedia.org/wiki/Chakra. Using the colors of the rainbow to represent each chakra came about in the 1970's. Lilly, S., & Lilly, S. (2003). Healing with crystals and chakra energies: How to harness the transforming powers of colour, crystals and your body's own subtle energies to increase health and wellbeing (p. 169). London, England: Hermes House. Vishnu-Devenanda, writing in 1960, assigns a different set of colors to the chakras. The two chakra color systems are described in the Appendix.

[32] Essential oil suggestions are from the Yoga Deck and from www.AuraCascia.com. See also http://www.auracacia.com/chakras/documents/aura-cacia-chakra-journey-ebook.pdf

[33] American Journal of Clinical Nutrition on June 26, 2013. First published June 26, 2013, doi: 10.3945/ajcn.113.064113. Am J Clin Nutr September 2013.

[34] For more on why we keep eating this garbage even when it doesn't taste good, see Haug, C. (2014) Rehab for Weight Loss, A Humorous Approach to Getting Skinny and Healthy [Kindle DX version]. Retrieved from Amazon.com.

[35] Mesko, p. 57.

[36] Miller, p. 14.

[37] Two brands of bath colors are made by Sesame Street and Crayola. The Crayola colors are richer and a little more expensive than Sesame Street.

[38] The Anjali mudra is also used as a gesture of reverence by holding our hands at our hearts or at our foreheads.

[39] Judith, p. 41.

[40] Miller, p. 22.

[41] McGonigal, K. (2012). The Willpower Instinct, How Self-Control Works, Why It Matters, and What You Can Do to Get More of It (pp. 147-148). New York, NY: Avery.

[42] Restore Your Health With Chakras, Pt 1 - The Secrets

In Your Chakras: Seven Energy Centers | The Dr. Oz Show. (n.d.). Retrieved from http://www.doctoroz.com/episode/secrets-your-chakras-7-energy-centers?video_id=2759276191001

43 Mesko, p. 112.

44 Not everyone can do a shoulder stand. So try the modified version which consists of lying on your back and bringing your knees to your chest.

[45] A Mudra for Vocal Empowerment. (n.d.). Retrieved from https://www.youtube.com/watch?v=9BtpRlomYEo   From the Aura Wellness Center. By Virginia Iversen, M.Ed .

[46] Judith, p. 69.

[47] Mercier, P. (2007). The Chakra Bible, The definitive guide to working with chakras (p. 267). London: Godsfield Press Ltd.

[48] Judith, p. 64-65.

[49] Miller, p. 38.

[50] Mesko, p. 130.

[51] Miller, p. 38.

[52] Find Chakra Balance Through Your Diet | The Oz Blog. (n.d.). Retrieved from http://blog.doctoroz.com/oz-experts/find-chakra-balance-through-your-diet

[53] Judith, p. 76.

[54] Find Chakra Balance Through Your Diet | The Oz Blog. (n.d.). Retrieved from http://blog.doctoroz.com/oz-experts/find-chakra-balance-through-your-diet.

[55] Miller, p. 44.

[56] Mesko, p. 146.

[57] Miller, p. 45.

[58] Find Chakra Balance Through Your Diet | The Oz Blog. (n.d.). Retrieved from http://blog.doctoroz.com/oz-

experts/find-chakra-balance-through-your-diet
[59] Namaste (pronounced nah-mahs-teh) means "The light in me honors the light in you" or "The divine in me honors the divine in you."

About the Author

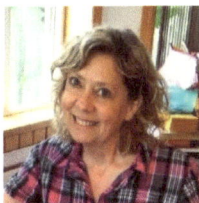

Cheri Haüg is a certified yoga instructor, weight loss coach and personal trainer. She teaches yoga in La Crosse, Wisconsin. She is the author of *Rehab for Weight Loss, A Humorous Approach to Getting Skinny and Healthy* available on Kindle and Nook. For more information, visit her website at www.ColorMyYoga.com.